1 Q From which regions of the central nervous system do parasympathetic nerves originate?	**2** Q From which regions of the central nervous system do sympathetic nerves originate?
3 Q What types of nerves arise from the spinal cord and innervate skeletal muscle directly?	**4** Q How many neurons are involved in parasympathetic transmission from the spinal cord to the target organ?
5 Q True or False? Craniosacral parasympathetic axons synapse on neurons in the peripheral ganglia.	**6** Q What neurotransmitter mediates parasympathetic nervous system function?
7 Q What neurotransmitter receptor mediates parasympathetic nervous system function at the peripheral ganglia?	**8** Q What neurotransmitter receptor mediates the parasympathetic tone in the cardiac muscle?

1. Cranial and sacral regions	2. Thoracic and lumbar regions
3. Somatic nerves	4. Two
5. TRUE	6. Acetylcholine
7. Nicotinic acetylcholine receptors	8. Muscarinic acetylcholine receptors (specifically M2)

9 Q What neurotransmitter receptor mediates the parasympathetic tone in the smooth muscle?

10 Q What neurotransmitter receptor mediates parasympathetic tone in the glandular cells?

11 Q Somatic nerves that arise from the spine innervate skeletal muscle. What neurotransmitter receptor, which is located on skeletal muscle, receives this input?

12 Q How many neurons are involved in sympathetic transmission from the spinal cord to the target organ?

13 Q Where is the first synapse after the spinal cord in sympathetic innervation of an organ?

14 Q True or False? Preganglionic sympathetic axons synapse on neurons in the peripheral ganglia.

15 Q At the paravertebral ganglia, the neurotransmitter _____ acts on _____ receptors to mediate sympathetic nervous system function.

16 Q What neurotransmitter mediates sympathetic nervous system function at the sweat glands?

9	10
Muscarinic acetylcholine receptors (specifically M3)	Muscarinic acetylcholine receptors (specifically M1 and M3)
11	12
Nicotinic acetylcholine receptors	Two
13	14
Preganglionic sympathetic axons synapse on neurons in the paravertebral ganglia	False preganglionic sympathetic axons synapse on neurons in the paravertebral ganglia
15	16
Acetylcholine nicotinic acetylcholine	Acetylcholine

17 Q	18 Q
What neurotransmitter receptor mediates sympathetic nervous system function at the sweat glands?	What neurotransmitter mediates sympathetic tone in the cardiac muscle, smooth muscle, and glandular cells?
19 Q	**20 Q**
What are four cell types in which α_1- and β_1-adrenergic receptors mediate sympathetic tone?	What neurotransmitter mediates sympathetic tone in the renal vascular smooth muscle?
21 Q	**22 Q**
What neurotransmitter receptor mediates the sympathetic tone in the renal vascular smooth muscle?	What two substances are released into the blood from the adrenal medulla after the activation of the sympathetic nervous system?
23 Q	**24 Q**
How many synapses are involved in activation of the adrenal medulla?	Are nicotinic acetylcholine receptors ligand-gated sodium-potassium channels or G-protein coupled receptors?

17	Muscarinic acetylcholine receptors	18	Norepinephrine
19	Cardiac muscle smooth muscle glandular cells and terminal ends of neurons	20	Dopamine
21	D1 receptors	22	Epinephrine and norepinephrine
23	One the adrenal medulla releases epinephrine and norepinephrine into the blood	24	Nicotinic receptors are ligand*gated sodium*potassium channels

25. Q Are muscarinic acetylcholine receptors ligand-gated sodium-potassium channels or G-protein-coupled receptors?

26. Q To what class of G-proteins is α,1-receptors linked?

27. Q To what class of G-proteins is α,2-receptors linked?

28. Q To what class of G-proteins is β,1-receptors linked?

29. Q To what class of G-proteins is β,2-receptors linked?

30. Q To what class of G-proteins is M1-receptors linked?

31. Q To what class of G-proteins is M2-receptors linked?

32. Q To what class of G-proteins is M3-receptors linked?

25 A	26 A
Muscarinic acetylcholine receptors are G*protein*coupled receptors that act through second messengers	q

27 A	28 A
i	s

29 A	30 A
s	q

31 A	32 A
i	q

33 Q	34 Q
To what class of G-proteins is D1-receptors linked?	To what class of G-proteins is D2-receptors linked?
35 Q	**36** Q
To what class of G-proteins is H1-receptors linked?	To what class of G-proteins is H2-receptors linked?
37 Q	**38** Q
To what class of G-proteins is V1-receptors linked?	To what class of G-proteins is V2-receptors linked?
39 Q	**40** Q
What are the major effects of α,1-receptor activation?	What are the major functions of α,2-receptor activation?

33 A	34 A
s	i
35 A	36 A
q	s
37 A	38 A
q	s
39 A	40 A
It increases vascular smooth muscle contraction and increases pupillary dilator muscle contraction (mydriasis)	It decreases sympathetic outflow and decreases insulin release

41. What are the major functions of β,1-receptor activation?	42. What is the major function of β,2-receptor activation on the body's vasculature?
43. What is the major function of β,2-receptor activation on the respiratory system?	44. What effect does β,2-receptor activation have on glucagon release?
45. Where are M1-receptors located?	46. What effect does M2-receptor activation have on cardiac function?
47. What are the effects of M3-receptor activation?	48. What effect does D1-receptor activation have on renal vasculature?

41 A	42 A
It increases heart rate and contractility increases renin release from the kidneys and increases lipolysis of adipose tissue	Vasodilation
43 A	**44** A
Bronchodilation	It increases glucagon release
45 A	**46** A
The central nervous system	It decreases heart rate and contractility
47 A	**48** A
Increased exocrine gland secretions gut peristalsis bladder contraction bronchoconstriction miosis and accommodation	It relaxes renal vascular smooth muscle

49 Q What are the effects of H1-receptor activation?

50 Q What is the effect of H2-receptor activation?

51 Q What effect does V1-receptor activation have on vascular smooth muscle?

52 Q The activation of what two types of G-protein-coupled receptors can increase vascular smooth muscle contraction? Which receptors mediate vascular relaxation?

53 Q What is the effect of V2-receptor activation? Where are they located?

54 Q What five types of receptors are coupled with Gq proteins?

55 Q What five types of receptors are coupled with Gs proteins?

56 Q What three types of receptors are coupled with Gi proteins?

49 A Pruritis pain nasal and bronchial mucus production contraction of bronchioles	**50** A It increases gastric acid secretion
51 A It increases vascular smooth muscle contraction	**52** A α1- and V1-receptors increase contraction, relaxation is mediated by β2, and D1(renal only)
53 A It increases water permeability and reabsorption in the collecting tubules of the kidney	**54** A α1, M1, M3, H1, and V1
55 A β1, β2, D1, H2, and V2	**56** A a2 M2 and D2

57 Q

What enzyme is activated directly downstream of Gq-coupled receptors?

58 Q

What enzyme is activated directly downstream of Gs-coupled receptors?

59 Q

What enzyme is inhibited directly downstream of Gi-coupled receptors?

60 Q

Adenyl cyclase catalyzes the conversion of adenosine triphosphate into what molecule?

61 Q

What final effector enzyme is activated by receptors that are coupled with Gs proteins?

62 Q

What final effector enzyme is inhibited by receptors that are coupled with Gi proteins?

63 Q

Phospholipase C catalyzes the cleavage of membrane lipids into what molecules?

64 Q

What is the effect of increased inositol triphosphate on the intracellular concentration of calcium?

57 A	58 A
Phospholipase C	Adenyl cyclase
59 A	60 A
Adenyl cyclase	cAMP
61 A	62 A
Protein kinase A	Protein kinase A
63 A	64 A
Inositol trisphosphate3 and diacylglycerol	It increases the intracellular calcium concentration

65 Q	66 Q
What enzyme is activated by diacylglycerol?	What pharmacologic agent blocks the uptake of choline into cholinergic nerve terminals?
67 Q	68 Q
What enzyme is responsible for the formation of acetylcholine? What are its two substrates?	What pharmacologic agent blocks the transport of acetylcholine into the presynaptic vesicles in nerve terminals?
69 Q	70 Q
The entry of what ion into the nerve terminal induces the release of acetylcholine into the synaptic cleft?	What toxin inhibits the calcium-induced release of acetylcholine from the cholinergic nerve terminals?
71 Q	72 Q
What enzyme breaks down acetylcholine in the synaptic cleft? What two products result from this reaction?	Tyrosine transporters are located in the nerve terminals of what type of cells?

65 A Protein kinase C	66 A Hemicholinium
67 A Choline acetyltransferase Acetyl*CoA and choline	68 A Vesamicol
69 A Calcium	70 A Botulinum
71 A Acetylcholinesterase choline and acetate	72 A Noradrenergic cells tyrosine is the precursor of norepinephrine

73 Q Tyrosine is a precursor to the formation of which neurotransmitters? What is the order of their synthesis?

74 Q What pharmacologic agent blocks the conversion of tyrosine to DOPA?

75 Q Tyrosine is converted into dopamine via what intermediate precursor?

76 Q What pharmacologic agent blocks the transport of dopamine into the presynaptic vesicles in nerve terminals?

77 Q Dopamine is converted into norepinephrine in the _____ (cytoplasm/presynaptic vesicle).

78 Q The entry of what ion into the nerve terminal induces the release of norepinephrine into the synaptic cleft?

79 Q What pharmacologic agent inhibits the calcium-induced release of norepinephrine from the noradrenergic nerve terminals?

80 Q What pharmacologic agent stimulates the release of norepinephrine from the noradrenergic nerve terminals?

73 A	74 A
Tyrosine DOPA dopamine norepinephrine epinephrine	Metyrosine

75 A	76 A
DOPA DOPA can be used as a pharmacologic agent to increase central nervous system dopamine	Reserpine

77 A	78 A
Presynaptic vesicles	Calcium

79 A	80 A
Guanethidine	Amphetamine

81 Q

How is norepinephrine cleared from the synaptic cleft?

82 Q

What pharmacologic agents inhibit the reuptake of norepinephrine into the nerve terminals?

83 Q

What three receptor types modulate the presynaptic release of norepinephrine from the noradrenergic nerve terminals?

84 Q

What effect does the activation of α_2-receptors in presynaptic sympathetic nerve terminals have on norepinephrine release?

85 Q

What effect does the activation of angiotensin II receptors in presynaptic sympathetic nerve terminals have on norepinephrine release?

86 Q

What effect does the activation of M2-receptors in presynaptic sympathetic nerve terminals have on norepinephrine release?

87 Q

The norepinephrine-mediated activation of α_2-receptors on presynaptic sympathetic nerve terminals is an example of a mechanism of what type of feedback?

88 Q

Name four direct cholinergic agonists.

81 — Diffusion metabolism (monoamine oxidase A) and reuptake	82 — Cocaine amphetamine and tricyclic antidepressants
83 — M2-receptors, angiotensin II receptors, and α2-receptors	84 — It inhibits norepinephrine release
85 — It stimulates norepinephrine release	86 — It inhibits norepinephrine release
87 — Negative feedback	88 — Bethanechol carbachol pilocarpine methacholine

89 Q	90 Q
What is the clinical application of bethanechol?	What is the mechanism of action of bethanechol?
91 Q	**92** Q
What two direct agonist cholinomimetic drugs can be used to treat glaucoma?	Carbachol and pilocarpine are effective for the treatment of open-angle glaucoma because they activate what muscle?
93 Q	**94** Q
What is a methacholine challenge test?	Pilocarpine is effective for the treatment of narrow-angle glaucoma because it activates what muscle?
95 Q	**96** Q
True or False? Pilocarpine is susceptible to acetylcholinesterase.	Name five indirect cholinergic agonists.

89 A	90 A
Treatment of postoperative and neurogenic ileus and urinary retention (remember: Beth Anne call (bethanechol) me if you want to activate your	Bethanechol is a direct cholinergic agonist resistant to acetylcholinesterase that works on receptors in the bowel and bladder
91 A	**92** A
Carbachol and pilocarpine	The ciliary muscle of the eye
93 A	**94** A
A test in which methacholine is inhaled to stimulate muscarinic receptors and induce bronchoconstriction to diagnose asthma	The pupillary sphincter
95 A	**96** A
False pilocarpine is resistant to acetylcholinesterase	Neostigmine pyridostigmine edrophonium physostigmine echothiophate

97 Q	98 Q
What are the clinical indications for the use of neostigmine?	True or False? The treatment of myasthenia gravis is a clinical application of pyridostigmine.
99 Q	**100** Q
Which anticholinesterase is used to diagnose myasthenia gravis? Why?	True or False? The treatment of glaucoma is a clinical application of physostigmine.
101 Q	**102** Q
Which pharmacologic agent is used to treat atropine overdose?	What is the clinical indication for use of echothiophate?
103 Q	**104** Q
Indirect cholinergic agonists increase endogenous acetylcholine by inhibiting what enzyme?	Why is pyridostigmine used to treat myasthenia gravis?

97 A	98 A
The treatment of postoperative and neurogenic ileus	TRUE

99 A	100 A
Edrophonium the effects last for minutes and if weakness is transiently reversed it is diagnostic of myasthenia gravis	True (remember: "PHYS is for the EYES")

101 A	102 A
Physostigmine because it crosses the blood*brain barrier and is able to reverse the central nervous system as well as peripheral nervous system	The treatment of glaucoma

103 A	104 A
Acetylcholinesterase	It increases the amount of acetylcholine in the neuromuscular synapse thereby increasing muscle strength

105 Q	106 Q
What effect does neostigmine have on the central nervous system?	What is the clinical application and mechanism of action of topical atropine, homatropine, and tropicamide?
107 Q	**108 Q**
What are the mechanism and clinical application for benztropine?	What are the mechanism and clinical application for scopolamine?
109 Q	**110 Q**
What are the mechanism and clinical application for ipratropium?	What are the mechanism and clinical application for methscopolamine?
111 Q	**112 Q**
What are the mechanism and clinical application for oxybutynin?	What are the mechanism and clinical application for glycopyrrolate?

105 A None it does not penetrate the blood*brain barrier (remember: NEO CNS = NO CNS)	**106** A These drugs antagonize muscarinic receptors in the eye to produce mydriasis and cycloplegia
107 A It is a muscarinic antagonist used to reduce symptoms of Parkinson's disease	**108** A It is a muscarinic antagonist used to treat motion sickness
109 A It is a muscarinic antagonist used to treat asthma and chronic obstructive pulmonary disease (remember: I PRAY I can breathe soon!)	**110** A It is a muscarinic antagonist used to treat peptic ulcers
111 A It is a muscarinic antagonist used to reduce urgency in mild cystitis and reduce bladder spasms	**112** A It is a muscarinic antagonist used to reduce urgency in mild cystitis and reduce bladder spasms

113 Q	114 Q
What are the mechanism and clinical application for pirenzepine?	What are the mechanism and clinical application for propantheline?

115 Q	116 Q
Which muscarinic antagonist can be used to reduce urgency in patients with mild cystitis?	Which muscarinic antagonist is most commonly used to treat motion sickness?

117 Q	118 Q
Which muscarinic antagonist can be used to treat bladder spasms?	You recently prescribed haloperidol to your patient to treat his schizophrenia, but he has since developed Parkinson's-like motor adverse effects. What drug could you add to his regimen to treat this?

119 Q	120 Q
Atropine is used for therapeutic effect in which four organ systems?	What are the two effects of atropine on the eye?

113 A	114 A
It is a muscarinic antagonist used to treat peptic ulcers	It is a muscarinic antagonist used to treat peptic ulcers
115 A	**116** A
Oxybutynin (also glycopyrrolate)	Scopolamine
117 A	**118** A
Oxybutynin (also glycopyrrolate)	Benztropine
119 A	**120** A
Eyes gastrointestinal system respiratory system urinary system	Pupil dilation cycloplegia

121 Q	122 Q
What is the effect of atropine on the airway mucosa?	What is the effect of atropine on the stomach?
123 Q	124 Q
What is the effect of atropine on gastrointestinal motility?	What is the effect of atropine on the bladder in a patient with cystitis?
125 Q	126 Q
(A) represents what neurotransmitter and receptor type?	Part of the sympathetic NS, sweat glands and adrenal medulla are innervated by which neurotransmitter/receptor group, marked (A) and (B)?
127 Q	128 Q
A patient affected by botulinum toxin will be affected at which neurotransmitter/receptor group(s)?	According to the mnemonic DUMBBELSS, what four major physiologic processes are blocked by atropine?

121 A	122 A
It decreases secretions	It decreases acid secretion

123 A	124 A
It decreases motility	It decreases urgency

125 A	126 A
Acetylcholine neurotransmitter nicotinic receptor	(A) acetylcholine neurotransmitter/muscarinic receptor (B) nicotinic neurotransmitter/muscarinic receptor

127 A	128 A
Botulinum toxin affects all neurotransmitter/receptor groups that have acetylcholine as the neurotransmitter	Diarrhea Urination Miosis Bronchospasm Bradycardia Excitation of skeletal muscle Lacrimation Sweating and Salivation

129 Q	130 Q
True or False? Increased body temperature is a sign of atropine toxicity.	True or False? Slower heart rate is a sign of atropine toxicity.
131 Q	132 Q
True or False? Dry mouth is a sign of atropine toxicity.	True or False? Dry, flushed skin is a sign of atropine toxicity.
133 Q	134 Q
True or False? Cycloplegia is a sign of atropine toxicity.	True or False? Diarrhea is a sign of atropine toxicity.
135 Q	136 Q
True or False? Disorientation is a sign of atropine toxicity.	Which two adverse effects of atropine are more common in elderly patients?

129 A	130 A
True (ie "hot as a hare")	False heart rate would be increased
131 A	132 A
True (ie "dry as a bone")	True (ie "dry as a bone red as a beet")
133 A	134 A
True (ie "blind as a bat")	False constipation is a sign of atropine toxicity
135 A	136 A
True (ie "mad as a hatter")	Urinary retention and acute angle closure glaucoma

137 Q

True or False? Atropine toxicity can cause urinary incontinence.

138 Q

True or False? Atropine toxicity can cause fecal incontinence.

139 Q

What type of acetylcholine receptors does hexamethonium antagonize?

140 Q

What effect does hexamethonium have on heart rate?

141 Q

Name four toxicities of hexamethonium.

142 Q

Name 11 drugs that act as direct sympathomimetics.

143 Q

Which types of receptors are activated by epinephrine?

144 Q

Low doses of epinephrine are selective for _____ (α_1, α_2, β_1, β_2) adrenergic receptors.

137 A

False atropine toxicity can cause urinary retention in men with prostatic hypertrophy

138 A

False atropine toxicity causes constipation not fecal incontinence

139 A

Nicotinic acetylcholine receptors

140 A

It can prevent bradycardia in response to increased blood pressure when pressors are given

141 A

Severe orthostatic hypotension blurred vision constipation sexual dysfunction

142 A

Isoproterenol dobutamine phenylephrine epinephrine norepinephrine dopamine albuterol terbutaline ritodrine metaproterenol and salmeterol

143 A

α1-, α2-, β1-, and β2-receptors

144 A

β1

145 Q

Which types of receptors are activated by norepinephrine?

146 Q

Does norepinephrine have a greater affinity for α,-adrenergic receptors or β,1-receptors?

147 Q

Isoproterenol is an agonist for which receptors?

148 Q

Which types of receptors does dopamine activate, and how strongly does it activate them relative to one another?

149 Q

Dopamine is an agonist for which receptors?

150 Q

Dopamine is _____ (ionotropic/not ionotropic) and _____ (chronotropic/not chronotropic), while dobutamine is _____ (ionotropic/not ionotropic) and _____ (chronotropic/not chronotropic).

151 Q

Phenylephrine is an agonist for which receptors?

152 Q

Metaproterenol, albuterol, salmeterol, and terbutaline are agonists for which receptors?

145 A	146 A
α1- and α2-, β1-receptors (with lower affinity)	α-Adrenergic receptors

147 A	148 A
β1- and β2-receptors equally	D1 = D2 receptors > β-receptors > α-receptors

149 A	150 A
β1- and β2-receptors	Ionotropic chronotropic ionotropic not chronotropic

151 A	152 A
α1-receptors > α2-receptors	β2-receptors > β1-receptors

153 Q

Ritodrine acts on _____ (α,1, α,2, β,1, β,2)-adrenergic receptors.

154 Q

What are the clinical applications of epinephrine?

155 Q

What effect does norepinephrine have on renal perfusion?

156 Q

What is the clinical application for isoproterenol?

157 Q

What role does dopamine have in treating shock?

158 Q

True or False? Dopamine can be used to treat heart failure.

159 Q

What are the clinical applications for dobutamine?

160 Q

What are the clinical applications of phenylephrine?

153 A	154 A
β2	Anaphylaxis open*angle glaucoma asthma hypotension
155 A	156 A
It decreases renal perfusion	Atrioventricular block
157 A	158 A
Increases blood pressure while maintaining renal perfusion	TRUE
159 A	160 A
Shock heart failure cardiac stress testing	Treats nasal decongestion causes vasoconstriction dilates pupils

161 Q	162 Q
What is the clinical application for albuterol?	Which sympathomimetics can be used to reduce premature uterine contractions?
163 Q	164 Q
Amphetamine, ephedrine, and cocaine are (direct/indirect) sympathomimetics.	By what mechanism does amphetamine exert its sympathomimetic effect?
165 Q	166 Q
By what mechanism does ephedrine exert its sympathomimetic effect?	By what mechanism does cocaine exert its sympathomimetic effect?
167 Q	168 Q
What are the clinical indications for the use of amphetamines?	What are the three clinical applications of ephedrine?

161 A	162 A
Acute asthma	Terbutaline salmeterol

163 A	164 A
Indirect	It stimulates the release of stored catecholamines

165 A	166 A
It stimulates the release of stored catecholamines	It inhibits catecholamine uptake in the nerve terminal

167 A	168 A
Narcolepsy obesity attention deficit hyperactivity disorder	To treat nasal congestion urinary incontinence and hypotension

169 Q	170 Q
True or False? Phenylephrine can be used to treat nasal congestion.	What are the effects of cocaine when used topically?
171 Q	172 Q
Is the effect of epinephrine on β,-receptors greater than, equal to, or less than its effect on α,-receptors?	Is the effect of isoproterenol on β,-receptors greater than, equal to, or less than its effect on α,-receptors?
173 Q	174 Q
What are the effects of norepinephrine on heart rate, systolic and diastolic blood pressure, and pulse pressure?	What are the effects of epinephrine on heart rate, systolic and diastolic blood pressure, and pulse pressure?
175 Q	176 Q
Why does norepinephrine administration result in reflex bradycardia?	Epinephrine causes an increase in heart rate via which receptor subtype?

169 A	170 A
TRUE	Vasoconstriction and local anesthesia
171 A Equal to, except at low doses, at which epinephrine is selective for β1	**172** A Greater than
173 A It increases systolic and diastolic blood pressure slightly increases pulse pressure (systolic increases more than diastolic) and reduces	**174** A It increases systolic blood pressure decreases diastolic blood pressure greatly increases pulse pressure and increases heart rate
175 A Norepinephrine raises blood pressure causing a vagal response that leads to reflex bradycardia via increased parasympathetic input to the heart	**176** A β1 receptors, although epinephrine exhibits affinity for both β subtypes, it is selective for β1 at low doses, leading to tachycardia

177 Q	178 Q
What effect does isoproterenol have on pulse pressure and heart rate?	What is the effect of clonidine on central adrenergic outflow? Which receptor does it act on?
179 Q	180 Q
What are the clinical applications of clonidine?	What is the effect of α_1-methyldopa on central adrenergic outflow? Which receptor does it act on?
181 Q	182 Q
What are the clinical applications of α_1-methyldopa?	What are two patient populations for which α_1-methyldopa is indicated (as an antihypertensive)?
183 Q	184 Q
What is the clinical application and mechanism of action of phenoxybenzamine?	Would you use phenoxybenzamine or phentolamine before removal of a pheochromocytoma? Why?

177 A	178 A
Increases pulse pressure and heart rate	It is an α2-agonist and decreases central adrenergic outflow, remember that the α2-receptor is responsible for negative feedback
179 A	180 A
Hypertension especially with renal disease because it does not decrease blood flow to the kidneys	It is an α2-agonist and decreases central adrenergic outflow
181 A	182 A
Hypertension especially with renal disease because it does not decrease blood flow to the kidneys	Renal failure patients pregnant patients
183 A	184 A
Phenoxybenzamine is a nonselective α-blocker that is used to treat pheochromocytoma	Phenoxybenzamine because it is irreversible. Phentolamine is reversible so the high levels of catecholamines released during surgery would

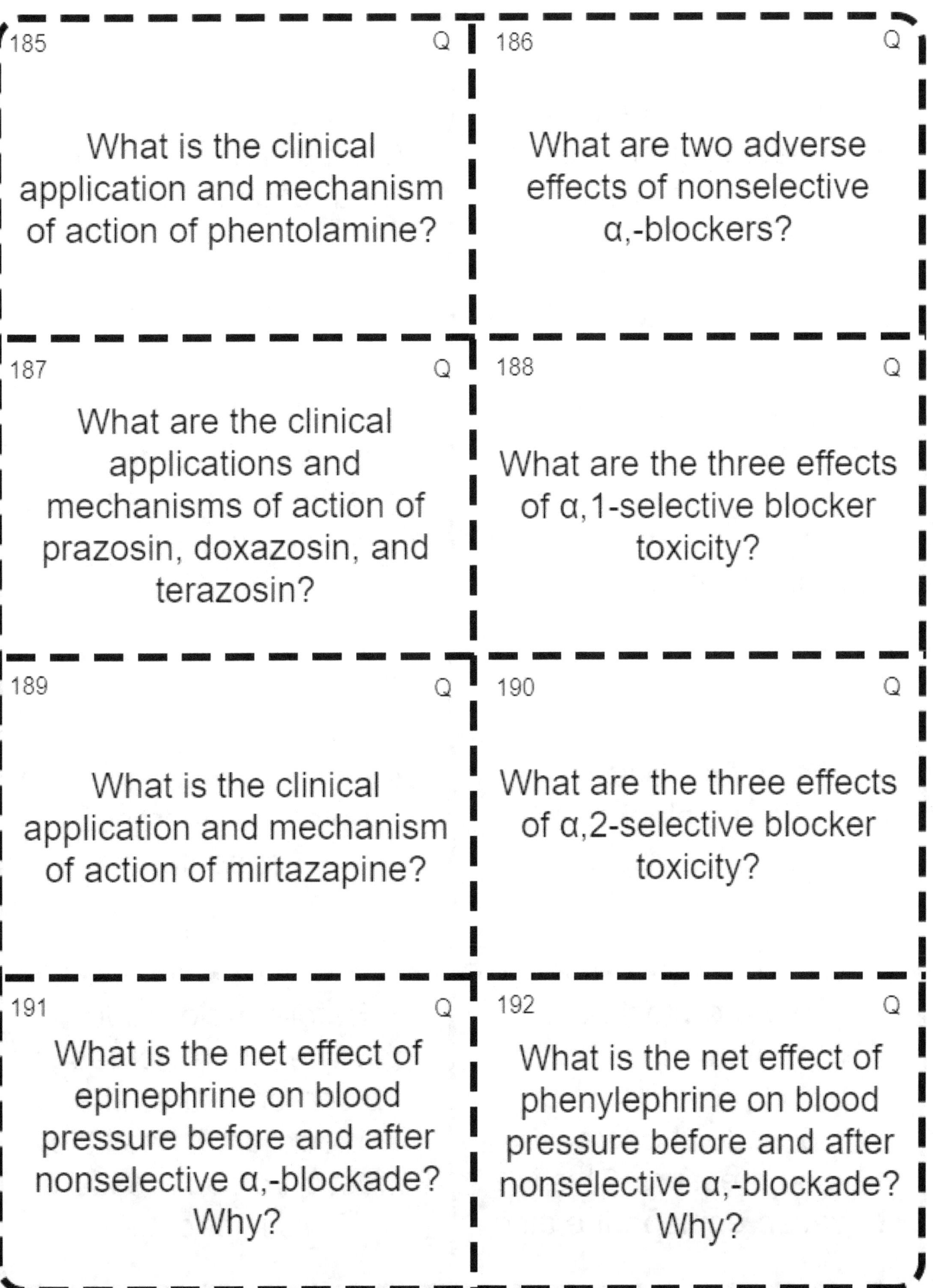

185 A	186 A
Phentolamine is a nonselective α-blocker that is used to treat pheochromocytoma	Orthostatic hypotension and reflex tachycardia
187 A	188 A
They are each an α1-selective blocker used to treat hypertension and urinary retention in benign prostatic hyperplasia	Orthostatic hypotension (first dose only) dizziness headache
189 A	190 A
Mirtazapine is an α2-selective blocker used to treat depression	Sedation increased serum cholesterol increased appetite
191 A	192 A
Before α-blockade, epinephrine increases blood pressure, after α-blockade, it decreases blood pressure. This is because epinephrine also	Before α-blockade, phenylephrine increases blood pressure, after α-blockade, it has little effect on blood pressure. This is because

193 Q

Why does epinephrine, a presser, cause hypotension if a patient is pretreated with an α₁-blocker?

194 Q

Name six clinical applications for β₁-blockers.

195 Q

Which two β₁-blockers are used to treat supraventricular tachycardia?

196 Q

What β₁-blocker is frequently used to treat glaucoma?

197 Q

How do β₁-blockers work in the setting of angina pectoris?

198 Q

A 63-year-old patient is referred to you from the emergency room for long-term care after his first myocardial infarction. Is a β₁-blocker suggested or contraindicated for this patient?

199 Q

What is the mechanism of β₁-blockers in the treatment of supraventricular tachycardia?

200 Q

To which class of antiarrhythmic agents do β₁-blockers belong?

193	If α-receptors are blocked, the β-agonist properties of epinephrine predominate and lower blood pressure
194	Hypertension angina pectoris myocardial infarction supraventricular tachycardia congestive heart failure glaucoma
195	Propranolol esmolol
196	Timolol
197	Decrease heart rate and contractility decrease myocardial oxygen consumption
198	Suggested after myocardial infarction patients should receive β*blockers to decrease the risk of mortality
199	They decrease atrioventricular conduction velocity
200	Class II drugs that slow atrioventricular conduction

201 Q	202 Q
How does the use of β,-blockers affect the progression of congestive heart failure?	What is the mechanism of β,-blockers in the treatment of glaucoma?
203 Q	204 Q
Why should β,-blockers be used with caution in diabetic patients?	Name five nonselective β,-blockers.
205 Q	206 Q
Name five β,1-selective antagonists.	Which β,-blocker is the shortest acting?
207 Q	208 Q
What β,-blockers have partial agonist activity?	What are two nonselective α,- and β,-antagonists?

201 A	202 A
Slows progression of heart failure, β-blockers reduce cardiac output but have proven benefit in congestive heart failure	They reduce the secretion of aqueous humor reducing intraocular pressure
203 A	204 A
β-Blockers should be used with caution in diabetic patients because they can block initial warning signs of hypoglycemia such as increased heart rate and	Propranolol timolol nadolol pindolol and labetalol
205 A	206 A
Acebutolol, Betaxolol, Esmolol, Atenolol, Metoprolol (remember: A BEAM of β1-blockers)	Esmolol
207 A	208 A
Pindolol, Acebutolol (remember: Partial Agonist)	Carvedilol labetalol

209 Q

A patient with a history of Graves' disease (hyperthyroidism) presents with chest pain. Her resting heart rate is 128 beats per minute, her blood pressure is 120/80 mmHg, and her respiratory rate is 18 breaths per minute. You order thyroid-stimulating hormone and thyroxine tests. What class of drugs would address her cardiac problems while you await the lab results?

210 Q

What is the mechanism of β_1-blockers in the treatment of hypertension?

211 Q

What are some effects of β_1-blocker toxicity?

212 Q

What symptoms indicate cholinesterase inhibitor poisoning?

213 Q

What mechanism underlies the symptoms of acetylcholinesterase inhibitor poisoning?

214 Q

The symptoms of parathion poisoning are caused by the inhibition of what enzyme?

215 Q

The symptoms of organophosphate poisoning are caused by the inhibition of what enzyme?

216 Q

A child ingests insecticide and presents with diarrhea, abdominal pain, wheezing, pinpoint pupils, and copious tears and salivation. What medication should he be given?

209 A ß-Blockers, such as propranolol, will reduce heart rate and consequently reduce angina	210 A Decreasing cardiac output and decreasing renin secretion
211 A Bradycardia atrioventricular block congestive heart failure (reduced cardiac output) sedation sleep alteration impotence exacerbation of	212 A DUMBBELSS: Diarrhea Urination Miosis Bronchospasm Bradycardia Excitation of the skeletal muscle and the central nervous system
213 A Inhibition of acetylcholinesterase leads to overactivity of the body's cholinergic systems	214 A Acetylcholinesterase
215 A Acetylcholinesterase	216 A Atropine and pralidoxime

217 Q

What antidote can be given to a patient who presents with diarrhea, urinary incontinence, miosis, bronchospasm, bradycardia, lacrimation, sweating, and salvation?

218 Q

Why is it important to give pralidoxime as well as atropine in organophosphate poisoning?

219 Q

Atropine is used as an antidote for what kind of poisoning? By what mechanism does it accomplish this?

220 Q

Pralidoxime is used as an antidote for what kind of poisoning? By what mechanism does it accomplish this?

221 Q

Penicillins are typically named with what suffix?

222 Q

Drugs used for the treatment of erectile dysfunction are typically named with what suffix?

223 Q

Drugs used for inhalational general anesthesia are typically named with what suffix?

224 Q

Phenothiazines are typically named with what suffix?

217 A

Atropine and pralidoxime

218 A

Because organophosphates are irreversible inhibitors of acetylcholinesterase and pralidoxime helps to regenerate functional

219 A

nophosphate/anticholinesterase inhibitor poisoning it inhibits muscarinic acetylcholine receptors

220 A

ganophosphate/cholinesterase inhibitor poisoning it regenerates active acetylcholinesterase

221 A

The suffix -cillin, such as methicillin

222 A

The suffix -afil, such as sildenafil

223 A

The suffix -ane, such as halothane

224 A

The suffix -azine, phenothiazines are neuroleptics such as chlorpromazine

225 Q	226 Q
Benzodiazepines are typically named with what suffix?	Antifungals are typically named with what suffix?

227 Q	228 Q
Some antibiotics that inhibit protein synthesis are named with what suffix?	Barbiturates are typically named with what suffix?

229 Q	230 Q
Drugs used for local anesthesia are typically named with what suffix?	Butyrophenones are typically named with what suffix?

231 Q	232 Q
Trichloroacetic acids are typically named with what suffix?	Protease inhibitors are typically named with what suffix?

225 A	226 A
The suffix -azepam, such as diazepam	The suffix -azole, such as ketoconazole
227 A	228 A
The suffix -cycline, such as tetracycline	The suffix -barbital, such as phenobarbital
229 A	230 A
The suffix -caine, such as lidocaine	The suffix -operidol, neuroleptics such as haloperidol
231 A	232 A
The suffix -ipramine, such as Imipramine	The suffix -navir, such as saquinavir

233 Q	234 Q
β,-Antagonists are typically named with what suffix?	Drugs that end in -azine are generally what class of drug?

235 Q	236 Q
Cardiac glycosides are typically named with what suffix?	Drugs that end in -azole are generally what class of drug?

237 Q	238 Q
Drugs that end in -barbital are generally what class of drug?	Drugs that end in -caine are generally what class of drug?

239 Q	240 Q
Drugs that end in -cillin are generally what class of drug?	Methylxanthines are typically named with what suffix?

233 A	234 A
The suffix -olol, such as propranolol	Phenothiazines (neuroleptics antiemetics)

235 A	236 A
The suffix -oxin, such as digoxin	Antifungals

237 A	238 A
Barbiturates	Local anesthetic

239 A	240 A
Penicillins	The suffix -phylline, such as theophylline

241 Q	242 Q
Drugs that end in -cycline are generally what class of drug?	Drugs that end in -ipramine are generally what class of drug?

243 Q	244 Q
Angiotensin-converting enzyme inhibitors are typically named with what suffix?	ß,2-Agonists are typically named with what suffix?

245 Q	246 Q
Drugs that end in -navir are generally what class of drug?	Drugs that end in -olol are generally what class of drug?

247 Q	248 Q
Drugs that end in -operidol are generally what class of drug?	Drugs that end in -oxin are generally what class of drug?

241 A	242 A
Antibiotic or protein synthesis inhibitors at the 30s subunit of the ribosome	Tricyclic antidepressants

243 A	244 A
The suffix -pril, such as captopril	The suffix -terol, such as albuterol

245 A	246 A
Protease inhibitors	β-Antagonists

247 A	248 A
Butyrophenones (neuroleptics)	Cardiac glycosides (inotropic agents)

249 Q	250 Q
H2-antagonists are typically named with what suffix?	Drugs that end in -phylline are generally what class of drug?

251 Q	252 Q
Drugs that end in -pril are generally what class of drug?	Pituitary hormones are typically named with what suffix?

253 Q	254 Q
Drugs that end in -terol are generally what class of drug?	Drugs that end in -tidine are generally what class of drug?

255 Q	256 Q
α,1-Antagonists are typically named with what suffix?	Drugs that end in -triptyline are generally what class of drug?

249　A	250　A
The suffix *tidine such as cimetidine	Methylxanthines

251　A	252　A
Angiotensin-converting enzyme inhibitors	The suffix *tropin such as somatotropin

253　A	254　A
β2-Agonists	Histamine2 antagonists

255　A	256　A
The suffix -zosin, such as prazosin	Tricyclic antidepressants

257. Drugs that end in -tropin are generally what class of drug?

258. Drugs that end in -zosin are generally what class of drug?

259. Drugs that end in -afil are generally used for what purpose?

260. Drugs that end in -ane are generally used for what purpose?

261. Drugs that end in -azepam are generally what class of drug?

262. In enzyme kinetics, competitive inhibitors _____ (resemble/do not resemble) the substrate while noncompetitive inhibitors _____ (resemble/do not resemble) the substrate.

263. In enzyme kinetics, the value of Km reflects the _____ of the enzyme for its substrate.

264. True or False? In enzyme kinetics, the lower the Km, the higher the affinity.

257 — Pituitary hormones	258 — α1-Antagonists
259 — Erectile dysfunction	260 — Inhalational general anesthesia
261 — Benzodiazepines	262 — Resemble do not resemble
263 — Affinity	264 — TRUE

265. In enzyme kinetics, Vmax is directly proportional to the _____ _____.

266. In enzyme kinetics, a graph of substrate concentration on the x-axis and velocity of the reaction on the y-axis has _____ (increasing/decreasing) velocity as the substrate is increased.

267. When velocity is equal to one half of its maximum (Vmax), the corresponding concentration of substrate is equal to what value?

268. In enzyme kinetics, the y-intercept of a graph that plots the inverse of velocity on the y-axis and the inverse of substrate concentration on the x-axis is equal to what value?

269. In enzyme kinetics, the x-intercept of a graph that plots the inverse of velocity on the y-axis and the inverse of substrate concentration on the x-axis is equal to what value?

270. In enzyme kinetics, the slope of a graph that plots the inverse of velocity on the y-axis and the inverse of substrate concentration on the x-axis is equal to what value?

271. In enzyme kinetics, a competitive inhibitor _____ (cannot/can) be overcome by increasing the concentration of substrate, a noncompetitive inhibitor _____ (cannot/can) be overcome by increasing the concentration of substrate.

272. In enzyme kinetics, competitive inhibitors _____ (increase/decrease/do not change) the Vmax of the reaction, while noncompetitive inhibitors _____ (increase/decrease/do not change the Vmax of the reaction.

| 265 | Enzyme concentration | 266 | Increasing although it will plateau when the enzyme is saturated |

| 267 | Km | 268 | The inverse of Vmax = 1/Vmax |

| 269 | The inverse of Km = 1/Km | 270 | Km/Vmax |

| 271 | Can cannot. This is because competitive inhibitors bind the active site of the enzyme competing with the substrate whereas | 272 | Do not change decrease |

273 Q

In enzyme kinetics, competitive inhibitors _____ (increase/decrease/do not change) the Km of the reaction, while noncompetitive inhibitors _____ (increase/decrease/do not change the Km of the reaction.

274 Q

What is the formula for calculating the volume of distribution of a drug?

275 Q

Drugs with a low volume of distribution, such as 4-8 L, are found in the _____ (blood/extracellular space/tissues).

276 Q

A drug with a volume of distribution of 15 L is most likely to be found in the _____ (blood/extracellular space/tissues).

277 Q

In a 75 kg man, a drug has a volume of distribution of 40 L. It can be expected to be found in _____ (blood/extracellular space/tissues).

278 Q

What is the formula for calculating the clearance of a drug?

279 Q

What is the definition of the half-life of a drug?

280 Q

How many half-lives of a drug must pass before a drug infused at a constant rate reaches approximately 94% of steady-state concentration?

273 A	274 A
Increase do not change	The volume of distribution = amount of drug in the body/plasma drug concentration
275 A	276 A
Blood alone these drugs do not distribute outside the plasma	Extracellular space these drugs distribute throughout the total body water
277 A	278 A
Tissues	Clearance (L/min) = rate of elimination of drug (g/min) / plasma drug concentration (g/L)
279 A	280 A
The time required to reduce the amount of drug in the body by one half	Four

281 Q Given the volume of distribution and clearance of a drug, how does one calculate the half-life of the drug?	**282** Q After one half-life, given a constant intravenous infusion of a drug, how close to steady-state is the concentration of the drug?
283 Q After three half-lives, given a constant intravenous infusion of a drug, how close to steady-state is the concentration of the drug?	**284** Q What is the formula for the loading dose of a drug?
285 Q What is the formula for a maintenance dose of a drug administered intravenously?	**286** Q How do loading and maintenance doses of drugs differ for patients with hepatic and renal disease?
287 Q What is the bioavailability of a drug if it is administered intravenously?	**288** Q In zero-order elimination of drugs from the body, what is the relationship between the rate of elimination and the drug concentration?

281 A Half*life = (0.7 × volume of distribution) / clearance	**282** A 50% of steady*state concentration
283 A 87.5% of steady*state concentration	**284** A Loading dose = (target plasma concentration × volume of distribution) / bioavailability
285 A Maintenance dose = rate of elimination/bioavailability = (target plasma concentration × clearance) / bioavailability	**286** A For both hepatic and renal disease loading dose does not change but maintenance dose decreases
287 A 1	**288** A The rate of elimination is constant regardless of drug concentration

289 Q

What are the three drugs that exhibit zero-order elimination?

290 Q

In first-order elimination of drugs from the body, what is the relationship between the rate of elimination and the drug concentration?

291 Q

In zero-order elimination of drugs from the body, how does the plasma concentration of a drug change over time: linearly or exponentially?

292 Q

In first-order elimination of drugs from the body, how does the plasma concentration of a drug change over time: linearly or exponentially?

293 Q

Weak acids get trapped in _____ (acidic/basic) environments.

294 Q

Weak bases get trapped in _____ (acidic/basic) environments.

295 Q

What substance is given to enhance the renal clearance of weakly acidic drugs such as phenobarbital, methotrexate, and aspirin?

296 Q

What substance is given to enhance the renal clearance of weakly basic drugs such as amphetamine?

289 A	290 A
Phenytoin and ethanol aspirin at toxic concentrations	The rate of elimination is directly proportional to the drug concentration a constant fraction (rather than a constant amount) is eliminated
291 A	292 A
Linearly	Exponentially
293 A	294 A
Basic	Acidic
295 A	296 A
Bicarbonate	Ammonium chloride

297 Q	298 Q
Ionized species become trapped in urine because they are not _____ _____.	A 24-year-old man attempts suicide by consuming a small bottle of aspirin. After three hours he thinks better of it and comes to the emergency room. He is put in your care, and you start him on intravenous saline with bicarbonate. By what mechanism does this help him?
299 Q	300 Q
What three types of biochemical reactions are involved in the phase I metabolism of drugs?	What is the polarity of the drug products that result from phase I metabolism?
301 Q	302 Q
True or False? Drug products that result from phase I metabolism are water soluble.	True or False? Drug products that result from phase I metabolism are often still active.
303 Q	304 Q
What enzyme system mediates the phase I metabolism of drugs in the body?	What three types of biochemical reactions are involved in the phase II metabolism of drugs?

297 A	298 A
Lipid soluble therefore they cannot cross cell membranes	Bicarbonate alkalinizes the lumen of his nephrons which traps acetylsalicylic acid within the lumen because it is a weak acid and is ionized in a basic

299 A	300 A
Reduction oxidation and hydrolysis	The products are slightly polar

301 A	302 A
TRUE	TRUE

303 A	304 A
Cytochrome P*450	Acetylation glucuronidation and sulfation these are conjugation reactions

305 Q

Do geriatric patients lose the ability for phase I or phase II drug metabolism first?

306 Q

Phase I metabolism of drugs yields _____ (nonpolar/slightly polar/very polar) molecules that are _____ (inactive/often still active), whereas phase II metabolism of drugs yields _____ (nonpolar/slightly polar/very polar) molecules that are _____ (inactive/often still active).

307 Q

The products of phase II metabolism of drugs are excreted by what organ?

308 Q

What is the definition of efficacy?

309 Q

What is the definition of potency?

310 Q

A drug that requires a very low dose to achieve its desired effect is considered _____.

311 Q

True or False? In pharmacodynamics, when a competitive antagonist is given, the maximal effect of an agonist is decreased regardless of how much additional agonist is given.

312 Q

What is the effect of a noncompetitive antagonist on the position of an agonist's dose-response curve?

305 A Phase I	306 A Slightly polar often still active very polar inactive
307 A Kidneys	308 A Maximal effect a drug can produce
309 A Amount of drug needed for a given effect	310 A Potent
311 A False the maximal effect of an agonist is still achievable in the presence of a competitive antagonist if increased amounts of the agonist are given	312 A It vertically shrinks the agonist's efficacy is decreased

313 Q

In pharmacodynamics, the addition of a noncompetitive agonist _____ (increases/decreases/does not change) the efficacy of the agonist.

314 Q

How does the efficacy of a partial agonist relate to the efficacy of a full agonist of the same receptor?

315 Q

How does the potency of a partial agonist relate to the potency of a full agonist of the same receptor?

316 Q

What property of a drug is determined by its therapeutic index?

317 Q

What is the formula that describes the therapeutic index of a drug?

318 Q

Safer drugs have _____ (higher/lower) therapeutic index values.

319 Q

What is the antidote for acetaminophen overdose?

320 Q

What are the two treatments for salicylate overdose?

313 — Decreases	314 — A partial agonist has lower maximal efficacy than a full agonist
315 — A partial agonist may be more potent than less potent than or equally as potent as a full agonist	316 — Safety drugs with higher therapeutic indices are less likely to cause toxicities
317 — TI (therapeutic index) = LD50 (median toxic dose) / ED50 (median effective dose) (remember: TILE)	318 — Higher
319 — N-acetylcysteine	320 — Alkalinization of urine and dialysis if necessary

321 Q	322 Q
What compound is used to alkalinize urine?	What is the treatment for amphetamine overdose?
323 Q	324 Q
Amphetamines are _____ (acidic/basic), therefore, overdose is treated with _____ (NH4Cl/NaHCO3) to _____ (acidify/alkalinize) the urine.	What are the two antidotes for anticholinesterase toxicity?
325 Q	326 Q
What are the antidotes for organophosphate poisoning?	What is the antidote for toxicity caused by anticholinergic agents?
327 Q	328 Q
Physostigmine is the antidote for toxicity caused by what two types of agents?	What is the antidote for β,-blocker toxicity?

321	322
NaHCO3 weak acids are better excreted when the urine is alkaline	NH4Cl

323	324
Basic NH4Cl acidify	Atropine to block cholinergic receptors and pralidoxime to regenerate acetylcholinesterase

325	326
Atropine and pralidoxime organophosphates inhibit acetylcholinesterase	Physostigmine it inhibits acetylcholinesterase increasing the available acetylcholine to overcome anticholinergic toxicity

327	328
Antimuscarinic agents and anticholinergic agents	Glucagon

329 Q

What are five treatments for digitalis toxicity?

330 Q

What is the antidote for iron toxicity?

331 Q

What are four treatments for lead poisoning?

332 Q

Penicillamine is the antidote for toxicity caused by what substances?

333 Q

What are three treatments for arsenic poisoning?

334 Q

What are two treatments for mercury poisoning?

335 Q

What are three treatments for gold poisoning?

336 Q

Dimercaprol and succimer are the antidotes for toxicity caused by what substances?

329 A	330 A
Stop the medication normalize the potassium level give the patient lidocaine give the patient anti*digoxigenin Fab fragments give the patient	Deferoxamine a chelating agent
331 A	332 A
Edetate calcium disodium dimercaprol succimer and penicillamine	Copper arsenic gold
333 A	334 A
Dimercaprol succimer penicillamine	Dimercaprol and succimer
335 A	336 A
Dimercaprol succimer penicillamine	Mercury arsenic gold

337 Q	338 Q
The combination of thiosulfate and nitrite is the antidote for toxicity caused by what substance?	Hydroxocobalamin is the antidote for toxicity caused by what substance?
339 Q	340 Q
What are the treatments for cyanide poisoning?	What is the treatment for methemoglobinemia?
341 Q	342 Q
Methylene blue is used to treat elevated serum levels of what substance?	What are the treatments for carbon monoxide poisoning?
343 Q	344 Q
What are the treatments for methanol and ethylene glycol (antifreeze) poisoning?	Fomepizole is an antidote for toxicity caused by what substances?

337 Cyanide	338 Cyanide
339 Hydroxocobalamin or a combination of nitrite and thiosulfate	340 Methylene blue vitamin C
341 Methemoglobin	342 100% oxygen and hyperbaric oxygen
343 Ethanol dialysis and fomepizole	344 Methanol ethylene glycol

345 Q	346 Q
What are the antidotes for opioid overdose?	Naloxone is the antidote for overdose of what substance?

347 Q	348 Q
What is the antidote for benzodiazepine overdose?	Flumazenil is the antidote for overdose of what substance?

349 Q	350 Q
What is the treatment for tricyclic antidepressant overdose?	Alkalinization of the serum with sodium bicarbonate is a treatment for an overdose with what class of antidepressant medications?

351 Q	352 Q
What is the reversal agent for heparin?	Protamine is used to reverse the effects of what pharmacologic agent?

345 A Naloxone or naltrexone	346 A Opioids
347 A Flumazenil, it reduces the action of benzodiazepines at γ-aminobutyric acid receptors	348 A Benzodiazepines
349 A Sodium bicarbonate it can prevent cardiac arrhythmias	350 A Tricyclic antidepressants the alkalinization can prevent cardiac arrhythmias
351 A Protamine	352 A Heparin, however, it does not reverse low-molecular-weight heparin

353 Q	354 Q
What agents are used to reversing the effects of warfarin?	Vitamin K is used to reverse the effects of what pharmacologic agent?
355 Q	**356** Q
What agent is used to reverse the effects of both tissue plasminogen activator and streptokinase?	Aminocaproic acid is used to reverse the effects of what two pharmacologic enzymes?
357 Q	**358** Q
What is the antidote for theophylline?	A woman brings her 3-year-old son to the emergency room because she found him eating pills out of the acetaminophen bottle. She is not sure how many he ate but says that the bottle was almost empty by the time she got to him and that he was eating them one hour ago. Which drug should be administered to minimize further liver toxicity?
359 Q	**360** Q
Which component of multivitamins is the most likely to cause fatal overdose in children?	What is the mechanism of cell death in iron poisoning?

353	A	354	A
Vitamin K and fresh frozen plasma		Warfarin	

355	A	356	A
Aminocaproic acid		Tissue plasminogen activator and streptokinase	

357	A	358	A
β-Blockers		N-acetylcysteine	

359	A	360	A
Iron		Peroxidation of membrane lipids	

361 Q	362 Q
What will a patient with acute iron poisoning present with?	After gastrointestinal bleeding in the acute phase of iron poisoning, what is the progression of the clinical presentation?
363 Q	364 Q
Which antidepressants can cause tachycardia due to anticholinergic action?	Which drugs can cause coronary vasospasm?
365 Q	366 Q
Which drugs can cause cutaneous flushing as an adverse effect?	Which drugs cause dilated cardiomyopathy?
367 Q	368 Q
Which drugs can cause torsades de pointes?	What cardiac adverse effect can result from either cocaine or sumatriptan use?

361 A	362 A
Gastric bleeding	Metabolic acidosis followed by gastrointestinal strictures and obstruction

363 A	364 A
Tricyclic antidepressants	Cocaine and sumatriptan

365 A	366 A
Vancomycin adenosine niacin calcium channel blockers (remember: VANC)	Doxorubicin (Adriamycin) daunorubicin

367 A	368 A
Class III (sotalol) and class IA (quinidine) antiarrhythmic agents cisapride	Coronary vasospasm

369 Q	370 Q
What is the major adverse effect of niacin use?	Which drugs can cause agranulocytosis as an adverse effect?
371 Q	372 Q
Which drugs (or exposures) can cause aplastic anemia as an adverse effect?	Which antihypertensive drug can cause hemolytic anemia?
373 Q	374 Q
Which antibiotic can cause "grey baby syndrome"?	Which drugs can cause hemolytic anemia in G6PD-deficient patients?
375 Q	376 Q
Which drugs can cause megaloblastic anemia?	What is the major adverse effect of oral contraceptives?

369	370
Flushing	Clozapine carbamazepine colchicine propylthiouracil methimazole

371	372
Chloramphenicol benzene nonsteroidal anti*inflammatory drugs propylthiouracil methimazole	α*Methyldopa

373	374
Chloramphenicol	Isoniazid Sulfonamides Primaquine Aspirin Ibuprofen Nitrofurantoin (remember: hemolysis IS PAIN)

375	376
Phenytoin Methotrexate Sulfa drugs (remember: Having a blast with PMS)	Thrombotic events such as deep vein thrombosis and pulmonary embolus

377 Q

Which antihypertensive drug can cause chronic cough?

378 Q

What is the advantage of angiotensin II receptor blockers (like losartan) over angiotensin-converting enzyme inhibitors?

379 Q

Which drugs can cause pulmonary fibrosis?

380 Q

What adverse effect would you suspect in a newly jaundiced patient recently started on azithromycin?

381 Q

Which drugs (or exposures) can cause hepatic necrosis?

382 Q

What effect can isoniazid have on the liver?

383 Q

Which drugs can cause pseudomembranous colitis?

384 Q

Administration of clindamycin or ampicillin can cause an overgrowth of which bacteria in the colon?

377	378
Angiotensin*converting enzyme inhibitors	Angiotensin II receptor blockers are often prescribed as an alternative renoprotective antihypertensive medication in patients with
379	380
Bleomycin busulfan amiodarone	Acute cholestatic hepatitis
381	382
Halothane valproic acid acetaminophen Amanita phalloides	Hepatitis
383	384
Clindamycin and ampicillin are commonly implicated but many antibiotics can be responsible	Clostridium difficile which leads to pseudomembranous colitis

385 Q	386 Q
What adverse effect occurs when exogenous glucocorticoids are rapidly withdrawn?	Which drugs are known to cause gynecomastia?
387 Q	388 Q
Which drugs can cause hot flashes?	Which drug can cause gingival hyperplasia?
389 Q	390 Q
Which drugs can cause gout?	Osteoporosis can be caused by long-term use of which drugs?
391 Q	392 Q
Which drugs induce photosensitivity?	Which drugs can cause Stevens-Johnson syndrome?

385. Adrenocortical insufficiency due to long-term hypothalamic-pituitary-adrenal axis suppression, this is why steroids are usually

386. Spironolactone Digitalis Cimetidine Alcohol (chronic use) estrogens Ketoconazole (remember: Some Drugs Create Awesome Knockers)

387. Tamoxifen clomiphene

388. Phenytoin

389. Furosemide and thiazide diuretics

390. Steroids heparin

391. Sulfonamides Amiodarone Tetracyclines (remember: SAT for a photo)

392. Ethosuximide lamotrigine carbamazepine phenobarbital phenytoin sulfa drugs penicillin allopurinol think anticonvulsants and

393 Q Which drugs can cause a lupus-like syndrome?	394 Q Which adverse effects of fluoroquinolones are specific to children?
395 Q Which drug can cause Fanconi's syndrome if taken after its expiration date?	396 Q Which drugs can cause interstitial nephritis?
397 Q Which two drugs can cause hemorrhagic cystitis?	398 Q Which drug is administered to prevent hemorrhagic cystitis from the use of ifosfamide or cyclophosphamide?
399 Q Name two drugs that can cause cinchonism.	400 Q Which adverse effect of lithium can cause hypernatremia?

393 A	394 A
Hydralazine Isoniazid Procainamide Phenytoin (remember: it's not HIPP to have lupus)	Tendonitis tendon rupture and cartilage damage
395 A	**396** A
Tetracycline	Methicillin nonsteroidal anti*inflammatory drugs and furosemide
397 A	**398** A
Cyclophosphamide and ifosfamide	Mesna
399 A	**400** A
Quinidine and quinine cinchonism describes headache and tinnitus	Diabetes insipidus

401 Q	402 Q
Name two drugs that can cause diabetes insipidus.	Name three drugs that can cause seizures.

403 Q	404 Q
Which class of drugs can result in tardive dyskinesia?	What drugs can cause a disulfiram-like reaction?

405 Q	406 Q
Polymyxins are toxic to which organ systems?	Which drugs can cause both ototoxicity and nephrotoxicity?

407 Q	408 Q
A 60-year-old man presents with sudden severe great toe pain. On microscopy, an aspirate of the joint shows crystals. His medications include daily baby aspirin, a thiazide diuretic to control hypertension, a ß₁-blocker to control a cardiac arrhythmia, and a nonsteroidal anti-inflammatory drug for joint pain. Which of these medications likely contributed to his presentation?	What are the seven most common drugs that induce cytochrome P450 enzyme activity?

401 A	402 A
Lithium and demeclocycline	Bupropion imipenem/cilastatin isoniazid

403 A	404 A
Antipsychotics	Metronidazole certain cephalosporins procarbazine first*generation sulfonylureas

405 A	406 A
Neural and renal as a result it is usually only used topically	Aminoglycosides vancomycin loop diuretics cisplatin

407 A	408 A
Thiazide diuretics	Quinidine Barbituates St. John's Wort Phenytoin Rifampin Griseofulvin Carbamazepine (remember: Queen Barb Steals Phen*Phen and

409 Q	410 Q
What are the six most common substances that inhibit cytochrome P450 enzyme activity?	Which drug can both induce and inhibit different forms of cytochrome P450 enzymes? Is induction or inhibition its more significant effect?
411 Q	412 Q
Ethylene glycol is converted to oxalic acid by which enzyme?	Alcohol dehydrogenase converts ethylene glycol into what?
413 Q	414 Q
What substance is converted to oxalic acid by alcohol dehydrogenase?	What are two adverse effects of oxalic acid?
415 Q	416 Q
What enzyme converts methanol to formaldehyde and formic acid?	What does alcohol dehydrogenase convert methanol into?

| 409 Sulfonamides Isoniazid Cimetidine Ketoconazole Erythromycin Grapefruit juice Acute alcohol use (remember: Inhibit yourself from drinking beer from a | 410 Quinidine induction is more significant |

| 411 Alcohol dehydrogenase | 412 Oxalic acid |

| 413 Ethylene glycol it is usually found in antifreeze | 414 Acidosis and nephrotoxicity oxalic acid crystallizes in the kidney to cause damage |

| 415 Alcohol dehydrogenase | 416 Formaldehyde and formic acid |

417 Q	418 Q
What are two adverse effects of formaldehyde and formic acid?	Alcohol dehydrogenase converts what alcohol into formaldehyde and formic acid? |//
419 Q	420 Q
What enzyme converts ethanol to acetaldehyde?	Acetaldehyde dehydrogenase converts what substrate into acetic acid?
421 Q	422 Q
What does alcohol dehydrogenase convert ethanol into?	What enzyme that is involved in ethanol metabolism is inhibited by disulfiram?
423 Q	424 Q
Ethanol competes with what endogenous hormone substrate for binding in renal tubules?	Alcohol dehydrogenase converts what alcohol into acetaldehyde?

417	Severe acidosis retinal damage	418	Methanol
419	Alcohol dehydrogenase	420	Acetaldehyde
421	Acetaldehyde	422	Acetaldehyde dehydrogenase
423	Antidiuretic hormone the result is a diuretic effect	424	Ethanol

425 Q	426 Q
What are the four adverse effects of acetaldehyde?	Alcohol dehydrogenase is involved in the metabolism of what three alcohols?
427 Q	**428 Q**
Alcohol dehydrogenase is inhibited by what drug?	Acetaldehyde dehydrogenase is inhibited by what drug?
429 Q	**430 Q**
What enzyme converts acetaldehyde to acetic acid?	What does acetaldehyde dehydrogenase convert acetaldehyde into?
431 Q	**432 Q**
Name the eight drugs that can cause allergic reactions in patients with known sulfa allergies.	What are some clinical manifestations of sulfa-allergic reactions?

425 A Nausea headache vomiting hypotension	**426** A Ethylene glycol methanol and ethanol
427 A Fomepizole the drug can be used to prevent toxicities of methanol and ethylene glycol ingestions	**428** A Disulfiram the drug worsens the adverse effects of alcohol use and is also called Antabuse
429 A Acetaldehyde dehydrogenase	**430** A Acetic acid
431 A Celecoxib probenecid furosemide thiazides methoprim/sulfamethoxazo sulfonylureas sulfasalazine and sumatriptan	**432** A Fever, pruritic rash, Stevens-Johnson syndrome, hemolytic anemia, thrombocytopenia, agranulocytosis, uriticaria

433 Q

A patient presents to the emergency room with a fever, intensely pruritic rash, and urticaria. You ask her what medications she is taking, and she replies, "I can't remember the names, but I just switched to a different type of diuretic." What is a possible drug-related cause of her symptoms?

433 A

She is allergic to sulfa drugs and was just switched to furosemide or a thiazide

www.ingramcontent.com/pod-product-compliance
Lightning Source LLC
Chambersburg PA
CBHW081006170526
45158CB00010B/2936